Uli Zar

Secret
of staying slim & healthy

A practical guide
to the fulfillment
of your body

To support organic farming

Contents

Acknowledgements

Many people have asked me to write a book about my experience and the knowledge I have gained over the years about nutrition and the simplicity of effectively losing weight, staying slim and being really healthy. At last I have done it!

My heartfelt thanks go to Kasia who helped me with so many aspects of writing this book, including the research. Without her bright mind, endless patience, insistence on accuracy and sheer hard work, I could never have done it.

Thanks also to Paul Roos who helped me to formulate ideas and put the words on paper. We spent many happy and interesting hours discussing nature, science, philosophy and so many other things.

Chapter 1

What inspired me to write this book?

Although I can think of quite a few reasons why I decided to write this book, for me one of them stands out like a lighthouse on a dark night.

We live in the twenty-first century where mind-blowing technological advances and modern marvels literally abound, and yet the incidence of obesity, cancer, heart disease and diabetes is not only on the increase, but reaching frightening, runaway proportions.

Despite the unprecedented increase in knowledge, more and more people are suffering from these and other disorders. Why?

Thinking about the last four decades of my life there have been so many startling discoveries and inventtions. From faster and better cars to faster and more athletic human beings breaking records one after the other. From simple, small, monochrome televisions to high resolution, high density flat screen TVs. Now, with computers, the internet and mobile phones just about any information is instantly available. You don't even need to leave your home to see historical events unfold in real time on the other side of the globe.

From manually cleaning your house with a feather duster and a broom, we now have the convenience of ultra-modern vacuum cleaners, dishwashers and washing machines, to name but a few.

From spending hours to prepare a meal, we now do it in minutes with microwave ovens and pre-prepared food. Life is so much easier than 40 years ago.

Most new technology is good but when it comes to nutrition, technology is not necessarily our friend. During the last 40 years, season in and season out, wild animals' food has not changed and they are generally as healthy as they have always been. We need to eat more fresh, live food and not more quick, ready, fast food which is certainly not good for us.

Forty years ago I discovered the secret to becoming and staying slim and healthy. This is my story.

As a fat young teenager I found it hard to accept my physical state. By the same token I find it hard to accept the large percentage of obese people in today's society. The reason is very simple: they are eating the wrong food. This book solves this mystery and provides the simple solution to this vexing problem.

I grew up in a very loving family. My mother loved cooking. She cooked every single day, and she put a lot of effort and passion into her cuisine. She made sure the food was delicious. She was filled with pride and delight when we licked the plates. She always cooked what we liked, and she invested much time and money in keeping our taste buds entertained.

Mother was always on the lookout for a new recipe and was not afraid to experiment and try out tasty new combinations. She was truly passionate about cooking.

She baked the most gorgeous cakes once or twice a week. As a result, our house always smelled nice and food was always a central part of our lives. When it came to food preparation, the meals were invariably elaborate, over-cooked, over-spiced, and contained too much of everything. Nevertheless, we enjoyed every bite and when mother encouraged us to have more we duly obliged.

My mother firmly believed that more food would ensure the health of her family: rather too much than too little. Mother herself was short of stature and heavy set and she weighed at least 100 kilograms (220 pounds), maybe even more.

When I was 16 years old I became uncomfortably aware that I was very fat while all my friends were slim and good-looking. I weighed about 75 kilograms (165 pounds). I discovered it was very difficult to buy clothes because my clothes could only be one shape: shapeless! In order to cover my bulging stomach, the garments were more like tents than dresses.

When I went shopping with my friends, I felt jealous of them because they could buy fashionable clothes while I could not. My clothes always had to be the same shape: somewhat loose and never tight because tight clothing would show how fat and out of shape I was.

My friends told me not to worry and that I simply had a big bone structure like my mother. Just accept it, they said, you are what you are. (If you meet me today, you'll see that I actually have a small bone structure.) I would never be slim, they said. But I didn't agree. Deep down in my heart, I knew I could be slimmer.

Even though my mother loved fashion, she always had to wear the same clothes with the same shape, because nothing else would fit. It cost her a lot of money too, because she could only buy clothes from the special shops that catered for overweight customers, or she would have clothes specially made to fit her bulky frame. She told me that not everybody could be slim. Some people simply were fat by nature, she said.

My father said I should be grateful that I was healthy. "Healthy people eat", he said, "And when you're sick you lie in hospital, and you have no appetite. Sick people do not eat." True enough, I suppose, but I wanted to be slim and trim. Thinking about it now, it's true that people who spend lengthy periods in hospital tend to lose weight.

I thought the solution would be easy. I would simply reduce the amount I ate at home. When mother cooked dinner I would eat only half a portion. But this resulted in me being permanently hungry and I started bingeing and eating junk food. I became stressed out and depressed, so I ate even more junk food.

I will never forget the one particular day my mother asked me to go buy a loaf of bread. I bought one and at the time I was so stressed and so angry with myself that I ate the whole loaf! My mother asked me: "Did you buy the loaf of bread, Uli?" I said yes. "So where is it?" I told her I had eaten it. She didn't believe me. How could I eat a whole loaf of bread? But I did. It wasn't difficult for me. I made sandwiches, and before I knew it, I had finished the entire loaf.

The more stressed I became, the more my weight went up. I became desperately depressed. Then I decided to stop eating completely. For two days I ate very little. By the third day I was so hungry that I ate even more than before. I told myself "next week, on

Monday, I will start on a proper diet." But because I was permanently hungry, it didn't work. It was extra difficult for me because at home there was always a lot of nice food available as well as the aromatic smells of cooking in the air. Everything looked and smelled delicious. Often I ate even when I didn't feel hungry, simply because I was so stressed – and when I ate it just felt so good! My stomach was becoming huge, but I could always comfort and calm myself with food.

I used to go to the nearby beaches with my friends. As I walked, the sweaty insides of my thighs rubbed together. It was very tough on me, seeing all those good-looking people with trendy bathing suits and beautiful bodies having a great time.

One day when I was on a train, a man stood up and offered me his seat because he thought I was pregnant. I was very embarrassed and although I didn't show it, I was deeply hurt and crying out for an answer.

I read a lot of magazines and books about diets and special pills and drinks you could buy at pharmacies. They all guaranteed that if you followed their advice you would become slim.

My inner conflict was that I wanted to lose weight, while staying and looking healthy, but I also wanted to eat whatever I chose so that I could feel satisfied. All of the popular diets of the day prohibited many things and they were driven by rules – take these pills, don't eat this, don't do that. I didn't like such restrictions, so I didn't try any of those diets. I wanted to be like so many other people who are naturally slim and have a nice figure, even though they eat whatever they like. I wanted to be free to eat everything and not to be forced to avoid certain foods for the rest of my life, because I loved food so much – as I do to this day. If you are under stress and you are subjected to stringent dietary restrictions, your stress levels just increase. And the immediate solution to stress is to eat. That's why you need to eat the right food. Bad food choices (like sugar) damage your body and cause your brain to function incorrectly. I still couldn't understand why my friends were eating what they liked and still stayed slim.

My friends told me I would never be thin. "Look, your family is fat," they said. Genetically speaking their argument was sound, I suppose, but for some reason I was convinced that my whole family was eating incorrectly. The truth is that my friends' families ate very simply compared to our family. The reason I was fat was because I ate the food that my parents liked and I had grown accustomed to their ways.

One day my life changed dramatically. I read about an experiment by a scientist who was breeding rats. He divided them into 50 groups and fed every group according to the different ways people were eating. Some were fed bread and cookies. Some ate tinned food. Some were given food that was cooked very thoroughly. Some were fed according to different national diets – Italian, Mexican, Spanish, and so on. After a few years, he noted that the one group that remained slim, healthy and vigorous was the group eating everything fresh and natural – fresh meat, fresh fish, fresh fruit, vegetables, eggs and milk. The internal organs of these rats were well-proportioned and healthy, unlike the other groups. So he concluded that what nature provides has to be the best food.

This particular article made a huge impression on me; it really got me thinking.

Around about the same time I also read that the average human stomach has a volume of 1.45 litres (about 2.5 pints). Imagine one and half litres of food in an ice cream container of that size; that is the capacity of the human stomach. Not big. My stomach was definitely bigger than that. I had made another huge discovery, so I decided to concentrate mainly on my stomach.

At school we are generally taught that fresh vegetables are much better than cooked vegetables. The same information is available in books and magazines. The heat of cooking destroys a lot of the good ingredients. Fresh vegetables are richer in minerals, vitamins and nutrients. It's general knowledge, really. This is crucial information!

I don't know if it was merely coincidence or a meaningful collaboration of circumstances, but I started moving in the direction of exclusively eating fresh food to see what would happen. And guess what: I started to lose weight! Also, I wasn't as incessantly hungry as I used to be. No more round-the-clock hunger. In the first week I lost some weight. In the second week I lost more, although not quite as much. But as long as I kept losing weight I was happy.

That was over 40 years ago. I still am on that simple, fresh food diet, and I am very healthy and very slim. Today nobody believes that I was ever fat; people are convinced that I am one of those 'lucky' people who are born slim and trim, and I can eat whatever I like.

Thinking back I now realize how close I was to developing a serious mental disorder like anorexia or bulimia, because I so desperately wanted to be thin like my friends. I wish I could show you my photos when I was 16 or 17 years old, but I destroyed them all because I suffered to look at them. If I knew then that I was going to write this book, I would have kept those photos as proof. When you look at me now, you see a petite woman. No one else in my family was petite. People say I am lucky, but am I really? The more I eat right and exercise, the luckier I get!

Maybe you have reached the point that you believe there is nothing you can do about being overweight. You've tried everything you can think of. Diets work for a while and then you simply regain all that weight again. Maybe you've had children and the pregnancy has destroyed your figure. Perhaps you have been overweight all your life...

I can assure you, if you're patient and willing to lose weight naturally, I guarantee you will be able to demonstrate your success with your own before-and-after photos if you follow my tips about diet, exercise and attitude. It is really not difficult and it requires just a little bit of dedication to begin with. It all starts in the mind. You have to start now. This diet will work for anybody!

In my experience, the biggest challenge in getting yourself into shape is your stomach area. Whether you are slim or fat, you have to concentrate on your stomach. The condition of your stomach is the main indicator of your overall health and fitness.

When I was fat, I could easily eat two litres of ice cream in one go. Fortunately, I realised that if I kept eating low-nutrient food that was rich in sugars, fats, and all kinds of artificial things, I would need a greater quantity of food, which obviously caused my stomach to expand. To change that situation I knew I would have to switch to high-nutrient food. With better nutrition I would eat less and less, and so the size of my stomach would slowly shrink.

Visualise the size of a 1.5 litre (2.5 pint) ice cream container. I use an ice cream container because a container that holds fluids would be larger, as fluids are less dense. Remember, it receives all the solids and liquids you consume. The moment you exceed that limit, your elastic stomach has to expand. Of course, your amazing body is designed to cope with the occasional stretch, but if you do it too often you are enlarging your stomach.

This takes time. Not just a week or a month. Believe me, it is very unhealthy, even dangerous, to lose huge amounts of weight in two weeks. For example, a loss of ten kilos in two weeks would be wrong. Your body would literally suffer stress and shock.

So, whenever I bought food I always asked myself: does Mother Nature produce this or not? Is this food produced in a factory? I started listening to my body for what it needed, refining and developing my personal food choices, and gradually I lost weight. Nobody helped me. Some people even discouraged me, saying I would never be thin and that I was just fooling myself. It took me many months to establish my preferences for fresh food, and it might not be easy for you to change what you're eating initially. But if you do, you will be surprised at how good it will make you feel.

Take your time. During the first few weeks it might be tough, but after the first month it will become easier. After the first year you will never look back. Now, for me, 40 years later, nothing could be easier. There are no rules and no restrictions; I can eat anything. But because I've tasted success and I've learnt how certain foods make me feel afterwards; I try to avoid them and I usually choose fresh fruit, vegetables, meat, fish, dairy products and eggs. Not quantity but quality.

While I was still fat and had already started eating fresh meat, vegetables and fruit, I ate only two or three times a day. My body seemed to require exactly the same amount of fruit, vegetables and meat every day. I also noticed that when I ate in the morning, I was somehow losing weight faster than when I ate at night. I remember a time when I would wake up very hungry at 4 or 5 o'clock in the morning. The hunger woke me. I went to the kitchen and ate a lot. I tried not eating after 6 o'clock in the evening. My weight was dropping – not very fast, but I was happy. It's important that you're not only slim, but also happy and healthy. You must enjoy your life.

People sometimes invite me to dinner (this is usually too late for me to eat) and I can eat food that is not my normal fare. I do this more to please the people who invite me than myself. Such a meal might leave my stomach feeling bloated, but I take it in my stride. It does not really affect me if it only happens occasionally.

In my twenties I was very healthy, with a strong immune system. I was hardly ever sick, regardless of how many sick people were around me. If things were very bad, I might pick up a cold for one or two days at most. My immunity was extremely good because I was eating proper food.

When people look at me now they say I am very lucky. I don't think I'm lucky. Some people say I must have an unusually good digestive system or good genes. But I reply that I exercise and I eat fresh food. That is the secret behind how I look and how I feel. It doesn't happen by accident. I tell them that I put some effort into how I look and anybody else can do the same. When I tell them that I eat a lot, they don't believe me. You can be 'lucky' too if you try my diet (when I say I eat a lot, I still keep my imaginary 1.5 litre ice cream container in mind to avoid expanding my stomach).

For the past 40 years my passion, perhaps even obsession, has been human biology and chemistry. I am tuned in to observing nature and applying these principles experimentally. That's why I know the value of exercising on an empty stomach, because that's what animals do: they hunt or forage for food when they are hungry.

Every single creature and organism in the universe has a specific diet. So many people get sick so often mainly because they are on the wrong diet. A diet that's right for you provides health, beauty, energy and a strong immune system. Animals know this instinctively.

I am a 60 year old woman. My clothes fit me exactly the same as when I was 25 years old. It is no coincidence at all. This is my diet. It's been a part of my life for four decades. I am very rarely sick. At my age I can genuinely compare myself favourably to most people in their twenties.

How about you?

You can find thousands of books on diets and food preparation in bookstores and some of them are very good. So why should you read my book? Because it contains the essential secret of permanent natural weight loss and with it you don't need any special knowledge of cooking methods. You need to understand that food preparation generally modifies the molecular structure of the food. The optimum nutrition is found in raw food. If you have to prepare it, I would prioritise the methods as follows: juicing, blending, steaming, cooking, baking, frying and microwaving. I don't recommend the last two methods at all.

Eating natural foods like fruit and vegetables is really very easy. Anyone can do it. As soon as you start slimming down and you see the improvements in your body and your complexion, as well as enjoying a boost of energy, you'll realise just how easy it is. Usually the only difficult part of this diet is to find the shops or markets that sell good quality fresh produce.

If I had access to this information as a young girl, more than 40 years ago, I could have saved myself a lot of trouble. But you have it right in front of you right now.

Have you ever wondered why more and more people are becoming obese in this modern age of medical, scientific and technological advances? The answer lies in our lifestyle and the type of food we consume. We have become lazy, overweight, stressed, sickly and depressed because we are simply not doing what our bodies were designed to do.

Physiologically we are no different to wild animals and yet, in terms of health and physical performance, we are so much worse off because we choose to ignore the most basic principles of nature.

In my opinion, based on four decades of experience, we have been incorrectly conditioned and indoctrinated... we lack basic knowledge. Because I struggled so much to lose weight, I made it my life's mission to find the simple solution that I am about to teach you.

None of us were born with a propensity to be fat. I know there are many who will disagree with me on this point. We can't control the size or the proportions of our bodies. We can't change our bone structure, for example, but we can control what we put in our stomachs.

Wild animals don't have the options that humans enjoy. They can't go to the shops and choose products. They live on food available to them and they are guided by instinct only. They hunt and forage when they are hungry and they eat natural food until they are satisfied.

Humans exercise their options based on conditioned tastes and traditions. Instead of eating apples they eat apple strudel. Please remember this example, because this is the very reason why so many people are obese. Apples are so much better for life and health than apple strudel.

Now here is the good news: you can stop counting calories and start eating fresh food – as much as you like. It's the 'unnatural' or 'dead' foods that make us fat and unhealthy: the sugar, processed flour, artificial spices, preservatives and condiments – to name but a few.

Our bodies ask for the nutrients that are found in fresh, live food. That's why we experience hunger. Most processed food lacks sufficient nutrients, causing us to get hungry again soon after eating a meal.

Nature has provided a vast array of nutrient rich foods for our benefit, full of the carbohydrates, proteins, vitamins, minerals and essential oils we need to function optimally. When we stuff our stomachs with foodstuffs lacking in nutrients, we are only fooling ourselves and getting fat and unhealthy in the process. Remember, an apple is less expensive than apple strudel, so you'll be saving money too!

Over the past 40 years I have been obsessed with researching food and I know for sure that counting calories has little or no value in the long run. What really matters is how fresh the food is that you eat. Fruit, for example, may have many more calories than rice cookies, but your body is far better off with the fruit. Your body wants nutrition from a natural product.

About 20 years ago I decided to start doing some exercise. Growing up I never liked exercising and I hated all forms of sport. Nevertheless, by studying animals and how effortlessly they achieve optimal physical appearance and performance, I realised that some form of exercise can be very beneficial. Reluctantly (at first) I started going to the gym.

I soon found out that by combining a fresh food diet with some exercise exponentially increases your ability to lose weight (or maintain weight) and also your ability to have a healthy, beautiful body. Exercise also lifts your mood, relieves stress and increases your energy levels.

So, to answer the question that I set out to answer at the beginning of this chapter, let me summarise my findings. After being hopelessly fat, unhealthy and depressed 40 years ago, I have found the perfect, effortless natural diet. I eat as much live food as I like and I never go hungry. By adding a simple exercise routine to my diet I believe I have attained an optimal healthy lifestyle. I have lots of energy, I am hardly ever sick, lazy or miserable. I have confidence in my appearance and I wear whatever I like. In short, I am happy and I enjoy my life.

Remember, stick to simple, fresh foods (organic if you can) and keep the volume of your stomach in mind. For even quicker results, although it's not essential, resolve not to eat after 6 pm in the evening.

Unlike other people, I don't spend hours in the kitchen preparing meals. Neither do I spend hours shopping for food. The time I save in this way I spend going to the gym or doing other things that I like.

This book is written to help you and it sets out to achieve and prove the following:

- Anyone can be slim.
- Your appearance is governed by what you eat.
- You can change your life with good food and exercise.
- You can make the right food choices all the time.
- As creatures of nature we must abide by natural principles.
- You can eat as much raw foods (like juices, smoothies and whole fruit or vegetables) as you like and you won't get fat.
- You never need to worry about food again or feel bad about making the occasional bad choice.
- You can save time and money by making good food choices.
- The time you save can be used for exercise or spending time with your loved ones.
- You can now stop searching for quick-fix diets.
- You can look good and enjoy life with a slim, healthy body.

- Try not to eat after 6 pm in the evening. This is not a must, but for the quickest results this works best.

I believe God wants us all to be healthy and slim and to enjoy our lives without unnecessary hardship. The challenge is for us to find the simple, natural ways to enable our bodies to do what they are designed to do. So let's do it!

Chapter 2

What does Mother Nature provide?

Mother Nature constantly and bountifully provides all the essential ingredients to sustain healthy life on Earth: sunshine, air, water and soil.

You have to understand nature first before you can apply its principles to your life; not only to lose weight, but to live a healthy life.

Plants, animals and humans all need the sun. Without exposure to sunshine for long periods of time people start feeling miserable, listless and irritable. When the sun comes out it brings a smile to our faces. The sun energises us and provides vitamin D, which is essential for life and good health.

Your body absorbs as much vitamin D from the sun as it needs. By taking steps to obstruct sunshine from reaching your skin you are robbing yourself of valuable vitamin D. Sun block lotions can actually be harmful to your health. Of course, you don't need to stay out in the sun until you burn – just a little common sense is needed. Everyone is different in this regard; you should know by now how much sunshine is adequate for your skin. Usually this depends on your skin type: the darker your skin, the more sun you need.

Fresh air is another essential ingredient to life, as we all know. Don't stay indoors all day long; take a walk and breathe in some fresh air. Even if you don't live near a beach, a forest or a mountain, the air outside is better than the air indoors. So give your lungs and your whole body a treat by regularly spending time outdoors. You will reduce stress and even improve your digestive system. This should be a daily routine, whether it's cold, warm or even rainy.

Water is truly a miracle of life. Its cleansing, refreshing and hydrating powers are peerless. You need to consume enough water, but not too much (about two litres a day). Excess water consumption can actually be harmful – more than three litres would be too much. I believe drinking freshly squeezed juice has much of the water you need, along with a host of beneficial nutrients. Most people don't drink enough water. Your body needs at least two litres of liquid every day.

Use water to cleanse and soothe your body. A strong shower is a great massage. Water also moisturises inhaled air and protects vital organs. It flushes the kidneys and liver enabling your body to get rid of toxins. It also softens the stool and speeds up the passage of waste through the intestines, simultaneously removing toxins.

Your entire body, most notably your blood, cells and your brain, consists of about 70 percent water. Research shows that a fluid needs to be modified or 'structured' before your body can use it. This modification process takes energy from your body. The structured water in fruit and vegetables is already modified, freeing up energy that your body can use to regenerate cells and fight disease. In other words, structured water provides energy and unstructured water takes energy. So drink enough fresh water, but consume fresh juices too, if you can, to find the optimum balance for your body. The water in fruit and vegetables is structured, making it ideal for easy use by your body's cells.

Soil is the foundation for all life on our planet. This complex material contains all the ingredients that are used as building blocks in our bodies. As a combination of minerals and organic matter it contains its own intricate ecosystem and collaborates with micro-organisms to naturally improve and replenish its own life-giving capacity. Along with the sun, water and fresh air, it can turn a tiny seed into a nourishing plant in an amazingly short period of time.

I have said all of this to make you realize that it is not just food, or a selection of food, that keeps you vibrant, happy and healthy. You need to interact with your environment and to correctly apply these vital elements. Give your mind a break from worry and tension by appreciating the beauty of nature and enjoying the many gifts that Mother Nature provides. If you wish to become and stay slim and healthy all your life, don't take these gifts for granted.

Just watch animals and learn from them. The first thing you'll notice is that they need no clothes. They are clad with feathers or fur and they seem to do just fine; they can generally stay in the sunshine without burning. In terms of food they take what is available to them: simple food that is in season. Where animals have to rely on their instinct, we humans are creatures of reason. To a large extent we have lost our instinctive ability.

Animals, for example, do not smoke or drink because their instinct does not call for it. We humans apply our reason – for better or for worse. Actually, humans have a huge advantage over animals because they have the capacity to solve just about any problem. However, if you compare the health and well-being of humans to that of most wild animals, you have to wonder. Because of their capacity to reason, humans are often presented with more than one option to solve a problem, and some of these options can be harmful.

Choosing the right food is absolutely vital. Animals, with their limited ability to choose, seem to be more successful than humans because their instinct leads them to simple, natural food options. People are more complex. Their needs differ. They have to use their ability to reason judiciously in order to make the correct nutritional choices.

When animals are pregnant they instinctively change their eating habits to facilitate the growth of a baby or babies in the womb. Their instinct is almost infallible.

Animals' instinct is geared towards sustaining and promoting life, whereas human beings use their reason for comfort and convenience. Animals generally do not abort their babies, for instance. If ever you thought wild animals can be cruel, think again. The cruelty committed by humans, invariably motivated by selfish reason, is far worse.

Female animals generally stay with their babies all the time during the first critical period of their lives, feeding, cleaning, warming and loving them. In days gone by human mothers would stay with their babies in the same bed for a whole month, properly bonding with the child. Today parents spend a lot of money on newborn babies, buying bottles, clothes, toys and so on, when all they really need is love and personal care. All of us need love more than material things.

We humans tend to over-complicate everything instead of choosing simple, natural options. Take breast-feeding for example: why feed a baby on an artificial milk formula if the mother has the very best natural food at her disposal? I think we should take another good look at nature; we can learn so much from its simple, efficient ways.

People also do not appreciate the enormously powerful ability of their own immune systems. Have you noticed how babies and toddlers will eat just about anything they find on the floor? Strangely enough, this hardly ever has detrimental effects. I believe this behaviour is necessary for their immune systems to get used to a hostile environment, and to build the capacity to resist bacterial threats.

Healthy people and healthy animals are not fat. This statement might startle some people, but it's a fact. By simply making the right choices and finding out how we as individuals fit into the natural scheme of things we can change our lives for the better. Only you can change your lifestyle. Only you have the power.

Usually, people are afraid to experiment. If they don't understand something they tend to stick with conventional wisdom. Who says the conventional wisdom is right? If something is not working, maybe you should try something else.

There are many ways to lose weight. If you eat only meat and fat, for example, you will be easily satiated and your stomach will shrink quite quickly. But is this diet healthy and sustainable? Will your body get all the nutrients it needs?

My favourite subjects at school were biology and chemistry, and they still are my favourites. I am fascinated by the perfect harmony found nature. Animals are born with just the right knowledge to survive and flourish. They know where to find their food and how much to eat. They don't have all the choices that we humans do; they can't go to shops and restaurants.

The members of the human race, of course, live in diverse circumstances. Some people live in warm climates, others inhabit colder climes. Some do more physical work than others. Many factors influence our choices, including traditions and beliefs. For that reason I believe that *no single diet* is good for all people. Because we are different, our bodies are different and we eat differently.

Seeing as we are all different, why should we eat the same food? Our bodies need the same nutrients, but as individuals we need those nutrients in different proportions.

How do we know what and how much to eat? The problem here is that we are exposed to too many opinions. The plethora of inconsistent information dumped on us by the media makes matters even worse.

When we feed our pets we often cause them to become overweight. That's because we have caused them to deviate from their ideal natural diet and lifestyle. Feed and treat a dog or a cat like their wild cousins in nature and they soon return to their perfect natural state. Pet dogs, for instance, can even develop diabetes when fed incorrectly.

It's the same with us. The trick is to find our most natural balanced diet. One way to find this balance is through experimentation, like I did 40 years ago. Fairly recently, new research has found that blood types are a reasonably good indicator of ideal food preferences. I have found this method to be about 70 to 80 percent correct.

According to this method people with blood type 'O', for example, have a preference for more meat in their diet. People with blood type 'A' are the opposite: they prefer more fruit and vegetables.

In nature, creatures feed on basically two types of food: vegetable matter and meat. A combination of these two types of food is all we need to survive and thrive. We have the same options as animals – these are the best food products we have. When we stray from the natural balance of foods that our bodies require, we start to need nutritional supplements.

You can study the blood type theory for yourself if you like, but you don't need to. You probably know many of your own food preferences already. If you listen to your body like animals do, with a little practice, you will know exactly what you should eat. Have you seen how pregnant women know instinctively, through their 'cravings', what their bodies need? If you eat something and don't feel good afterwards, you know it's not for you. Some people love avocado, for example, yet others have an allergic reaction to it.

If your body wants meat, don't fill yourself up with pasta. It may satisfy your immediate hunger, but it won't provide the nutrients your body was asking for. Did nature provide pasta? Of course not!

Whatever your blood type you should eat fresh food products. Fresh is best! We know that. Food must be alive and not dead. Cooking usually kills the nutrients in fresh food. Studies have also shown that microwave cooking also destroys nutrients. Remember the scientific experiment with the rats? You can thrive on fresh food and even heal your diseases by eating food as fresh as possible.

I have heard it said that eating microwave cooked food is one of the best ways to slowly kill yourself. In fact, everybody I know who regularly microwaves food has a weak immune system and they don't know why. This little oven literally kills the nutrients in your food.

Fresh food is always the right choice for your body. By sticking to a regimen of fresh food *you cannot get fat*. Fresh foods contain the right nutrients that will satisfy your hunger and correctly nourish your body. If you are always hungry, your body is crying out for fresh, nutrient rich food. Humans don't produce their own vitamin C, like some animals; that's why we need to eat different kinds of fresh produce.

Many people are obsessed with ready or partially ready foods. They spend hours shopping for food and they usually buy too much. A lot of it eventually finds its way into the rubbish bin. In the developed world tons of food is wasted daily. People buy lots of food just in case they might get hungry… Of course, big business caters for these impulsive food shoppers with fancy new packaging, new product offers and new taste experiences.

So often I see young children (around one year old) being fed sweets, savouries and cookies by their generally overweight mothers. These mothers think their kids love this food, even though they have no choice in the matter. This is where many of our nutritional and health problems begin. Children are incorrectly fed by their mothers.

This bad start in life can lead to illnesses like diabetes and, of course, obesity – along with a whole range of associated health problems. This is not a problem caused by genetics, it's a problem caused by ignorance. The wrong food makes you fat.

If we had a diet that we knew would satisfy our hunger and keep us healthy and slim, we would buy less and throw away less food (if you have bought too much fruit or vegetables, make juice or smoothies that are easy to consume). We would save money on 'fancy food', medicine and visits to the doctor. Is this starting to make sense to you yet?

You have a phenomenal body. Start off by dining on good quality fresh foods. See what works best for you. Learn to listen to your body. How do you feel after eating a certain type of food? Are you bloated or do you feel lethargic? Pay attention to the signals sent by your body. Soon you will simply ignore the ideas of most doctors and nutritionists because they don't know you or your own very unique and personal preferences. You will eat as much and as often as you like (while obeying these nutritional principles), never go hungry, look great and feel on top of the world!

At this point I would just like to say a few words to vegetarians who claim that eating meat is immoral. As an animal lover myself I hate the very idea of trophy hunting. But breeding animals for food has been an integral part of human history for thousands of years. No factory or laboratory can produce the kind of food produced by a plant or an animal. Mother Nature is without equal.

In nature animals eat animals. Whether you like it or not, we are a part of the same circle of life. I have noted that these very same holier-than-thou vegetarians have no qualms about wearing leather shoes or carrying leather handbags. Some animals are slaughtered only for their hides, like snakes and crocodiles.

I am not saying you should eat meat. By all means, if you can get by with fruit and vegetables go right ahead. Like I said previously, some people naturally prefer a vegetable-dominant diet. Others don't. In my experience people who do a lot of hard, physical work cannot survive without the unique proteins found in meat.

When it comes to meat, however, I have a problem with chicken. We all know that most chickens are raised in dreadful circumstances and boosted with hormones, steroids and antibiotics. Profit margins on chickens are small due to the very competitive market, so farmers are compelled to grow them as quickly as possible.

My advice is that if you don't know for sure that chickens are fed and kept properly, even though the packaging makes claims like "free range", be very careful. Chicken meat also goes 'off' very soon and can make you very sick.

You might say I have a very active imagination, but I have noticed what regular chicken-eating people look like: they look like chickens! The protruding belly and buttocks with the skinny legs is a dead give-away. I ask them: do you like chicken? They always say: I love chicken!

Everything you read in this book is a product of my passion for healthy living over the past 40 years. I have conducted my own research and investigated just about every idea I've come across. I have done extensive experiments and questioned many people about food and lifestyle choices.

I am not a doctor or a nutritionist. Frankly, I think that counts in my favour. My thinking has not been shaped by the pharmaceutical industry, the medical fraternity or the food business. All that matters to me is results. I have always wanted to stay slim and healthy. I have no hidden agendas.

My information is based on real life experience. Nutrition has always been my passion – some might even call it an obsession. Through observation and experiments on myself, my family and my friends over 40 years I now know, without a shadow of a doubt, that my methods work.

I genuinely wish I could take a hold of every human being on earth and "re-programme" his or her mind in terms of natural nutrition. Obesity, disease and mental disorders like depression would soon become very scarce. Obviously every person has the gift of free will, but I am convinced that I could make everyone slim and healthy. Wouldn't the world be a much better place?

If you really want to be slim, good-looking and healthy inside and out, follow my advice. I've seen it work in my life and in the lives of many others. My methods will works for anybody.

Watching an old French movie from the 1970s the other day, I noticed that women were built quite differently in those days. Even though they did not have the skinny look of today's actresses, with a thin layer of fat under their skins, their bodies were firm, slim and healthy. They looked great in my opinion, because they probably ate better than most women do today.

You will probably have pre-conceived ideas and notions because of articles you've read or advice you've been given. I cannot change your mind or argue with you on these issues. It's for you to decide.

It is my desire for people to slowly but surely change their thinking about nutrition.

There is no doubt in my mind that incorrect nutrition plays a huge part in causing disease. This results in a visit to the doctor who simply gives the patient pills that invariably only treat the symptoms and have a long list of damaging side effects. The pills actually prolong the duration of the disorder. The downward spiral has begun. There is a better way to be healthy: eat right to live right.

Should you take vitamin supplements? There is a lot of conflicting information on this issue. People often buy multi-vitamin supplements because they know they don't eat enough nutrient rich natural food. However, there are a number of studies proving that certain vitamin tablets go straight through your digestive tract without being absorbed. A plumber once told me that he has found many undigested pills in the sewage. Is this a case of money down the drain?

Do wild animals normally need vitamin supplements? No, of course not, because their natural diet adequately meets their nutrition needs. Fresh food, dear reader, is always the best option.

Pets can be given vitamin supplements in moderation because their food is not always nutritionally adequate. The same applies to humans. Moderation is the key; we don't live on vitamin supplements, we live on fresh food.

I have also met several overweight people who claim they are happy to be fat. But if you study them closely, you will find they suffer from various ailments and their so-called happiness is usually just false bravado. They generally also suffer from a lack of energy and they are permanently hungry because their bodies are asking for real nutrients.

These days you can order fast food by phone or the internet. Junk food is just a call or a click away. And yet your hunger soon returns after a meal of processed or unnatural foods. If your body gets what it really wants you will be satisfied and you won't crave 'stupid' food.

Healthy people have good appetites, but people often eat more than they need to, especially over weekends and holidays. When they meet up with friends and family their nutritional sense goes out the window. Overindulging on food, especially the wrong food, makes you lazy. People generally have more energy on a Friday than they do on a Monday.

Once you are settled into this beneficial eating pattern you will be surprised by how little you are really eating in an entire day. This never ceases to amaze me. Remember, I'm the girl who ate a whole loaf of bread in one sitting! When you are eating the right food, you can rely on your body to tell you when, how often and how much you should eat.

By adding a simple exercise routine to your lifestyle, like wild animals do all the time, you can maximise your health and your sense of well being – not to mention a beautiful body as an added bonus. I meet many different people in the gym. I once met an overweight lady who was struggling to do the prescribed weight-loss exercises. One day I said to her if we could exchange bodies for six months she would soon see a massive difference. Enthusiastically she said she'd love to have a slim body so that she could buy all the nice clothes and pretty outfits that she'd always dreamed about. Then I said for six months she would have to take very good care of my body and not drink sweet, fizzy drinks or alcohol, and no chips, sweets or processed food. Her eyes got bigger and bigger when I explained the requirements and she meekly said she liked to drink wine with her dinner and she loves fast food because it is very tasty. However, I could clearly see she was not prepared to change her bad eating habits.

Here is a great tip that you should commit to memory: when you go to a restaurant visualise the entire meal you are about to eat (and drink) fitting into a 1.5 litre container. Anything more will expand your stomach and make you feel uncomfortable. If you know the amount you can eat and you make sure you eat good, nutritious food you cannot fail. Use this method instead of counting calories. It is much more effective.

Remember, simplicity is always the best policy. The same goes for many other things in life like decorating your house or choosing clothes. Keep it simple! By simple I mean a fresh apple is first choice, its juice is second choice and so on. Apple strudel would be the last choice.

Over the years most of us have been programmed to enjoy complicated meals – as opposed to simple meals. We have to renew our way of thinking. It may look hard to do, but it is certainly not impossible.

If strawberries are in season, for example, and they are readily available in your area, eat as many strawberries as you like: breakfast, lunch and dinner. The berries are now at their best. Eat them whole, blend or juice them, whatever you like.

As I've said a few times before, each one of us is different. Once you've lost the excess weight you carried by eating fresh, natural food only, you can experiment a little. If you then settle for a regimen of say 70 percent high quality natural food and 30 percent 'less healthy' food, you will probably be able to keep your weight stable and stay healthy. However, you will have to discipline yourself very carefully to stick to this ratio. Only you know how good you are at self discipline.

Here are some interesting facts about the direct connection between food, our energy levels and our frame of mind. Although the brain weighs only two percent of our body weight, it uses the energy of 20 percent of our food intake when it is in a calm state, according to medical science. When it is stressed it uses up to fifty percent of the available food energy. When you are stressed, you are more prone to hunger pangs and binge eating (especially comfort foods containing sugar). This results in your stomach feeling uncomfortable and generally feeling lazy and sleepy. In the morning you wake up tired and this pattern develops into a destructive daily cycle.

If we put the wrong kind of food in our stomachs, it robs us of energy and indirectly causes stress.

Experiments with leading athletes in training have proved that over-processed foods cause them to steadily lose their normal energy levels. After about a week of regularly eating sweets and junk food while in training, they feel completely depleted, tired and lethargic.

I can tell you why this happens. If you regularly eat the right food (fresh and natural) you will have much more available energy at your disposal, allowing your body to feed your brain properly and not get lazy and tired. The correct diet will also melt away the excess fat on your body and make you feel more confident and less stressed. I strongly recommend you start with something like celery, carrot and apple juice to boost your energy levels.

What about dairy products? Again, some people thrive on dairy and others don't. Some are lactose intolerant. However, milk, cream, butter and cheese are good natural foods, packed with nutrients. Yoghurt and kefir are excellent because they effectively supplement and boost the beneficial bacteria in your digestive system. Kefir is lactose free, so it is ideal for those who shy away from dairy products. Home-made kefir and yoghurt is best; it is really hard to find all-natural versions of these foods in the food stores. Homemade is always best.

On the subject of yoghurt, there is very little decent yoghurt to be found in the food stores. Good yoghurt should at least include these types of bacteria: *Lactococcus acidophilus, Streptococcus thermophilus,* as well as other *lactobacilli* and *bifidobacteria.* Store-bought yoghurt usually contains stabilisers, modified bacteria and flavouring agents, which I don't particularly like – I prefer it to be as natural as possible. Always read the labels when you are in the food store.

What about eggs? Eggs are nature's miracle food. They have an astonishing list of nutrients and gram for gram probably the best quality protein available. New studies show that soft-boiled eggs or even raw eggs are healthier than the scrambled or fried versions. Make eggs a part of your daily diet!

By the way, just about all animals like eggs, even goldfish and lovebirds. Always follow nature; animals know the best products on the market!

What about sugar? Cane sugar is one of our worst enemies. It is extremely addictive. Without realising it most people are hopelessly addicted to sugar. It causes havoc on our natural blood sugar levels and can directly or indirectly lead to a long list of diseases. Sugar and processed foods like white flour are not called 'white death' for nothing. Sugar also acidifies your body, encouraging inflammation and creating the perfect environment for numerous diseases. Sugar also feeds destructive organisms in your body like *Candida* yeast, and it also encourages the growth of tumours. By consuming the natural sugars in fruit and vegetables, especially by juicing, you can satisfy or still sugar cravings. I know its hard, especially if you have been treated to sugar since you were a child, but if you can avoid sugar, you have won half the battle.

What about salt? Our bodies need salt, but regular white table salt is not good for you. It has been bleached and heated at extremely high temperatures and it usually contains an unhealthy additive to keep it from clogging. White table salt also often contains tiny pieces of quartz sand that are as sharp as broken glass and can scratch the inside of your intestines, causing inflammation. Good quality natural sea salt or rock salt (sold as Himalayan salt in some countries) is worth the extra cost. In most instances salted snacks like chips or pretzels have been flavoured with regular white table salt.

Nutrition is an art that can be learned. Use nature as your example and you can't really go wrong. Teach yourself to find the right balance of fresh, natural food that works best for your body. If you need to, have yourself tested for allergies to give you a better idea of the right types of food for your body. Do the same for your children and give them a valuable head start in life.

Ideally, we need a large range of natural products to fully satisfy all our nutritional needs and to keep our diets varied and interesting. Our menus should be as colourful as the rainbow. Buying fresh produce in season always makes nutritional and economical sense. Wild animals naturally eat food in season. Local food should also be your first choice.

If meat works well with your constitution, however, go ahead and eat meat. Again, raw meat, like steak tartare, is best, but you need to buy it from a trustworthy butcher. Cooked meat should never be over-cooked. Processed meats are bad for you.

Some people regularly experience headaches. Usually the reason is not enough fresh water, too much dairy products and meat, and too little fresh fruit and vegetables. Sugar and alcohol are also major culprits. You can minimise your headaches by changing your diet. Just try it and see what works for you. Exercise and more fresh air will also make a huge difference. In my experience a lot of water during exercise is great for reducing or eliminating headaches.

Do wild animals suffer from depression? No, not unless they are removed from their natural environment or contained in confined spaces like cages. Captive elephants have been known to cry real tears for no apparent reason. Animals in their natural state are generally quite happy. Humans are similar in that the happiest humans are the ones that live the most natural lifestyle. Fishermen, foresters and active farmers are known to have very little depression. Inhabitants of remote islands who eat simple food and live simple lives are living proof. With the right food and the right amount of exercise humans invariably tend to be happier and healthier.

If we constantly inhabit "boxes" like our homes and our offices, without adequate movement, sunshine and fresh air, we will naturally become depressed like caged wild animals. According to research the people who suffer from depression most are those who work on computers and also mechanics who work in workshops. Depression is not something out of the blue – there is a natural reason for it.

Everything that is produced by nature, if used correctly, is good for you. Animals have that good sense instinctively; we need to follow their example. We are prone to trusting doctors and pharmacists – maybe we should pay more attention to nature.

In summary then:
- Expose yourself to sunshine regularly.
- Breathe as much fresh air as you can.
- Drink at least two litres of liquid every day.
- Keep tabs on the volume of food in your stomach – no more than 1.5 litres.
- Check your blood group and find out if you comply with the blood group theory regarding food preferences.
- Avoid sugar, white flour, chicken (if not organic) and too many vitamin and mineral supplements.

- Don't be fooled by counting calories; it's about quality, not quantity.
- Avoid microwave-cooked food.
- Try to avoid regular, white table salt.
- If, for example, 70% of your diet consists of good natural foods and 30% consists of bad choices (processed food), you are still eating healthily.
- If you can learn to walk and talk and drive a car, you can learn to follow a natural, healthy, fresh food diet.

In your mind's eye see yourself slim and healthy. If you can believe it, you can achieve it!

* * *

"Vitality and beauty are gifts of Nature for those who live according to its laws". *Leonardo Da Vinci*

Chapter 3

What is the best way to condition and relax your body?

I would like to start this chapter with a brief illustration of myself when I was a child. When we played outdoor team games at school, I was always the last person to get selected for a team. Nobody wanted me, because I was fat, slow and not very nimble. I was a liability to the team.

Today I go to the gym every day of the week. It's hard to believe that the cumbersome little girl whom nobody wanted in their team now spends between half an hour and two-and-a-half hours daily doing exercises. How is that possible?

For me it's the feeling I get when I've finished a good stint in the gym. My body feels alive, my mind is alert, and I feel a wonderful sense of satisfaction and accomplishment.

Believe me, I am not a sporty person – I never have been and I never will be. But for the last 20 years of my life I have discovered the sheer joy of using my body for the purpose it was designed for.

Along with my eating plan it ensures my optimum health and keeps me in peak physical condition. I look good, I feel good and I'm up for any challenge that life can throw at me.

Some people take pills just to get by because it's easy and simple, but I eat right and exercise to make the most of my life. If we compare ourselves to animals, as I always do to find the right answers, this makes a lot of sense. Wild animals need to be active in order to eat. Some need to walk to find better grazing, some need to fly around to catch insects and others need to hunt their prey. All of them are motivated by hunger to get going. They have to be active if they want to eat.

This is a secret that I would like you to grasp and take to heart: hunger is a great motivator! I wish some people would refrain from eating unless they did some exercise. So, if they are lazy they would pine away from starvation. Moreover, when you are hungry from not having eaten for a few hours, your body will function at its best during exercise. In fact, in my experience and in the experience of others, this is the very best time to do something physical.

Many people eat before exercise, thinking that they will be weak if they don't. This is wrong! Exercising on an empty stomach will not harm you or impair your level of performance. On the contrary, your body functions at its best in these circumstances. Take a tip from nature and try it for yourself.

By all means, drink water before, during and after exercise. My own preference is for warm water with some fresh lemon before exercise and cold water with lemon juice afterwards (if I have lemons at home). You need to be hydrated to replace the fluids you lose during exertion. But don't eat until after you have finished. Simple food and good hydration are keys to a flat stomach.

In my experience going to the gym has the best lasting effects. The stimulation you get from interacting with other people has a lot to do with it. Trying to do exercise all on your own is hard to sustain and takes a lot of discipline.

There are two main types of exercise in the gym namely cardiovascular training and weight training. Some people prefer one or the other, depending on their goals, although many like to do a combination of both.

The best type of exercise for you probably depends on your body type. If you are more sturdily built, the chances are you'll probably prefer weight training. If you have a lighter build, you'll probably prefer more cardiovascular training. Of course, like animals, not all of us are the same. So choose the type of exercise that you like and do it regularly. That's the best way to start.

If you want to be slim and healthy and you want to get to your optimum state of wellness, you need to eat right and exercise. The two go together naturally. Eating the wrong food will invariably cause you to lose energy. By just eating right, like I did for 20 years (in those days gyms were not popular unless you were a serious sportsperson), your progress will be a lot slower, but you will lose weight and become healthier. However, the process is accelerated exponentially when you exercise as well, and you will experience a deep sense of satisfaction that is hard to explain in words.

In my case I like to exercise on an empty stomach in the morning, although you could do it in the afternoon after work if it suits you better. After my workout I have my first meal of the day and I eat as much as I want (within reason and without expanding my stomach), as long as I'm eating good quality food as discussed in the previous chapter. This routine charges me up with energy for the rest of the day.

Talking about routine, if you persist with a set of actions for 21 days, you will establish a new habit. Once you are in the habit of exercising it becomes routine, just like brushing your teeth every day. Before I go to bed at night I like to pack my clothes and get my gym bag ready for the next day, so there's no excuse to procrastinate. You should be ready to go.

If you prefer to exercise in the afternoon, I suggest you do so after you haven't eaten for a few hours. This principle might seem very simple to you, but it is very important. You'll notice that once you start exercising the hunger will disappear. After your workout the hunger will reappear and you can sit down to a most enjoyable meal.

Two periods of time are proven to be best for exercising: around sunrise and sunset. Obviously, you don't have to adhere to this precisely, but it is a good principle to keep in mind when planning your exercise schedule. Find a time that suits you best.

In our modern day lives we tend to have sedentary lifestyles; sitting behind a desk, on a couch or behind the steering wheel of a car. Our bodies don't even do a fraction of the work that they are supposed to do. No wonder we generally experience a subconscious state of frustration due to this inactivity. In addition, our muscles become weak. Layers of fat accumulate on our bodies because we consume much more fuel than we need for our meagre performance.

This sedentary type of lifestyle, coupled with bad eating habits, lead to your body being more susceptible to disease. Your immune system will not be as strong as it should be, and it won't be able to cope with bacteria, viruses and infections that are part and parcel of our environment. As a result you will probably be a regular visitor to the doctor and the pharmacy. You will probably feel tired during the day, struggle to concentrate properly and your energy levels will be at a low ebb.

If this is true in your life, you are a prime candidate for chronic disease, depression and even mental disorders. To combat these ailments you will probably take a range of medication – which invariably has a long list of damaging side-effects – and you may even resort to artificial means of escaping the stress and depression like developing a drinking habit.

By embarking on a regular exercise routine, you will literally feel years younger and your life will become so good that you'll wake up with a smile on your face every morning! If you would like to enjoy this type of feeling, you need to start exercising regularly today.

Wild animals have no option but to be active and eat the right food. Human beings have free choice, so it is up to us to make that decision and to stick with it.

What's the use of having the gift of free choice and superior intelligence if we don't use it to our advantage?

I have not had weight problems for many years, yet I stick to my eating and exercising routine because it infuses me with energy and confidence.

I have been on holidays in the past where I didn't go to the gym for a while and when I came back it was a struggle initially to get back into my old routine. But I stick to it because it refreshes me inside and out, and I can't imagine living life again without energy and vigour. Many people live life with hardly any energy.

To be perfectly honest with you, after all these years I still don't enjoy exercise. I see other people at the gym who relish physical activity – they really love it. But I don't. For me it's hard work. However, the part I love is the sheer exhilarating feeling I get once I've completed my workout and the abundance of energy I have on tap for the rest of the day. No pills can give you this feeling. The effects of medication are always temporary. I have had this marvellous feeling for over 20 years – can you imagine how happy I am?

People call me lucky or they think I live on nothing but carrots and water, but they are so wrong. I work hard at my exercise and I eat more than many people I know. The difference is that I eat the right kind of food. I try to minimise sugar, carbohydrates and foods with gluten.

You can do the same. Everybody likes energetic, healthy and happy individuals. Who wants to hang around tired, obese, sick and depressed people?

Do you remember the type of energy you had as a child? Well, you can have it again, no matter what your age. You can also have that same sharp, enquiring mind you had as child. You can have a bounce in your step and a grin on your face all the time. You can wear the clothes you really like and even flaunt the latest fashion. Trust me, when you are in shape you will really enjoy your own body. Would you like that?

I've had this discussion with many people. Some respond positively and others don't. Some people are seemingly content with the downward slide of ill health, constant tiredness and the onset of chronic disorders for example high blood pressure, diabetes and osteoporosis. They seem content to be overweight and permanently tired. They trundle back to the doctor month after month to collect more pills. Invariably they tell me they don't have time to exercise.

Let me share another secret with you: everybody on this planet has 24 hours every day. If something is important enough to you, you will find the time to do it. Your health should be your top priority, so don't tell me you can't do it. Some of the busiest executives in the world make time for exercise – that is why they can keep up with their busy schedules. And that is why they are successful. You don't have to be a sporty person to do some basic exercises every day. All you need to do is to make a decision. You have to look after yourself first to be strong in your mind.

Exercise also helps to get rid of the stress and the pent-up emotions that we all accumulate in life. The harder you exercise, the more stress you get rid of. Some people have a few drinks every day to get rid of their stress, but the next day they feel the damaging after-effects of the alcohol which causes them to get stressed out even sooner. Can you see the destructive cycle forming in this behaviour? Would you like to change? Start today!

Regular exercise promotes deep, relaxing sleep every night. I am so used to sleeping well that I am amazed at how people struggle with this basic necessity of life. Do animals have sleep problems? Sleep is a natural process for all species. If you have to take sleeping pills or alcohol to fall asleep, something is drastically wrong. Your body needs sleep to repair itself and to regenerate your cells. If you sleep well, the chances are good that you have a strong immune system and a healthy body.

Exercise gives you confidence and a great outlook on life. It might be a cliché but it's true: a healthy body houses a healthy mind.

You could say that a hundred years ago people didn't exercise and they were fine. But then in those days people walked a lot and they chopped wood and they did many physical chores. Also, most people didn't have refrigerators so they had to go to the market to buy fresh food and fresh milk almost every day. If they didn't go, they couldn't eat. If you don't work you shouldn't eat either. They ate much less processed food and hardly any food with preservatives. Treats like sweets and sugar were a rarity. In those days very few people were obese.

In some rural societies in faraway places like the South Sea Islands, people still hunt or fish for their food. They gather wood for their fires and they plant fresh vegetables or pick berries and fruit. None of them are obese or depressed. They sing and dance a lot. Diseases like cancer, diabetes or heart disorders are virtually unheard of in these societies. They might be poor by our standards, but they are healthy and happy.

Obesity has become commonplace in modern society, especially in the more developed countries. You really don't need a doctor or a nutritionist to tell you why. Just walk into a supermarket and see the type of food people are putting into their shopping trolleys. Just take a sneak peak at their inactive lifestyles and you'll know why they are fat.

If you want to be in peak physical health you need to eat the right food, do some exercise, sleep well and find ways to relax. All these things come naturally to wild animals. We humans can take charge of our lives and our bodies by learning from them.

Do I need to say anything more to motivate you? Anyone can change his or her life for the better, no matter how big or small or rich or poor you are. A journey of a thousand miles always starts with the first step, so take that first step today. Even if it means a 15 minute walk every day for a few weeks so that you can get fit enough for more demanding exercise later on.

If you take my advice today, I guarantee you will thank me profusely in a few short months from now.

Sleep

Sleep is by far the best form of relaxation. The deeper you can sleep, the better. However, some people need more sleep than others, because they don't sleep so deeply. It doesn't really matter if you're a day person or a night person, you need to be refreshed and revitalised when you wake up.

People who struggle to sleep well are often too stressed. Stress is a state of mind. Once you get into a good exercise routine you start looking forward to it every day – like a holiday. Your mind is occupied with good thoughts instead of bad thoughts. This will cause you to sleep a lot better. Sleeping well rejuvenates your body and your mind; you actually produce and release good, healthy hormones during deep sleep. Every species of animal on this planet needs to sleep properly to stay healthy and maintain a strong immune system.

Massage

A good massage can also cause you to be so relaxed that you feel drowsy and sleepy. This is a powerful relaxation technique.

Personally, I have one massage session a week. Afterwards I feel pleasantly relaxed, fall asleep quickly and I sleep a lot better. Sleeping well generates energy for the next day. In my experience you have to find the right masseur and you may need to experiment a little.

Massage also relieves the muscular stress you accumulate at work. Whether you sit behind a desk for hours or you lean over a dental patient all day long, a good deep-tissue massage can work the stress out of your tired muscles.

Just like food and exercise go together, so too massage and exercise work together to get rid of muscular tension.

Yoga

Yoga is also a superb method to relax your mind and body. It increases flexibility, improves your ability to breathe properly, stimulates and refreshes your mental capacity and it reduces stress.

Deep Breathing

With the focus on full, cleansing breaths, deep breathing is a simple yet powerful relaxation technique. It's easy to learn, can be practiced almost anywhere, and provides a quick way to get your stress levels in check. All you really need is a few minutes and a place to stretch out.

The key to deep breathing is to breathe deeply from the abdomen, getting as much fresh air as possible in your lungs. When you take deep breaths from the abdomen, rather than shallow breaths from your upper chest, you inhale more oxygen. The more oxygen you get, the less tense, short of breath, and anxious you feel.

- Sit comfortably with your back straight. Put one hand on your chest and the other on your stomach.
- Breathe in through your nose. The hand on your stomach should rise. The hand on your chest should move very little.

- Exhale through your mouth, pushing out with pressure as much air as you can while contracting your abdominal muscles. The hand on your stomach should move in as you exhale, but your other hand should move very little.
- Continue to breathe in through your nose and out through your mouth. Try to inhale enough so that your lower abdomen rises and falls. Count slowly as you exhale, as far as you can go.

If you find it difficult breathing from your abdomen while sitting up, try lying on your back. Put a small book on your stomach, and try to breathe so that the book rises as you inhale and falls as you exhale. You will also find this is a wonderful method to fall asleep when you have insomnia.

- Exercise at least five times a week.
- Don't eat before you exercise.
- Drink water before and after exercise (try it with some lemon).
- Choose the type of exercise you enjoy most.
- A sauna and steam bath can also be very beneficial and helps to detoxify your whole body.
- Always get enough sleep.

- A good massage works wonders (try to get one at least once a month).
- Yoga and deep breathing are also excellent for relaxation.

These simple principles are all guaranteed to improve your energy levels, promote a sense of well-being and they will greatly enhance the quality of your life.

Chapter 4

What is "super fuel" for your body?

All living plants are amazing miracles of nature. My own personal favourite plant is *hemp*. You may be surprised by this because a lot of misinformation has been communicated about this truly astonishing plant.

Where I grew up in Europe the farmers would plant hemp to feed their livestock during winter when the fields would be covered with snow. They knew this was the best food for their animals and they knew it kept them healthy in the cold months.

It has also been found that birds lay more eggs when they feed on hemp seeds.

New studies have shown that this plant has remarkable properties. For many years we have known that hemp produces the strongest natural fibre on earth, so it was previously used extensively to produce rope. But today we also know that it has significant nutritional and medicinal value. The seeds have an incredibly high protein content and they also contain probably the best balance of essential fatty acids known to man.

Today modern man mismanages the soil by over-using it and treating it with chemicals that unsettle the natural structure and balance of organisms in the soil. The result is that the soil cannot replenish itself the way nature intended and we are stuck with a growing medium that is nutrient poor.

As a result our farmers produce food that is also low in nutrients. Humans who eat the low-nutrient food that is made from these plants suffer from nutrient deficiencies which lead to ill health and other problems. In years gone by the food we harvested from the soil was certainly more packed with nutrients than it is today.

All living organisms need the correct amount and balance of nutrients to be able to grow and to be healthy. That is why I like to buy food products that have been organically produced. One of them is hemp seed and hemp seed oil. As a car needs good fuel to run the engine, so your body needs good fuel to function at its best.

Hemp seeds contain 30 to 35 percent high quality oil. The seeds are muscle builders and energy boosters of note, and in my opinion one of the most underrated sources of fuel for your body. This ancient food can be traced back thousands of years to the Chinese, Egyptian and Persian dynasties, when this plant was revered as a complete food source.

Hemp seeds contain an impressive list of amino acids and fatty acids and is being rediscovered as a complete food source high in energy, protein, dietary fibre and important minerals like magnesium. By including these seeds (shelled or unshelled) into your daily diet you can also expect to be hunger free for much longer. The seeds are a good source of GLA (Gamma Linolenic Acid) and natural CLA (Conjugated Linolenic Acid) which can assist in weight loss if consumed as part of a diet designed to assist in doing so.

Hemp seed oil is a natural product, which has ideal proportions, particularly important in the metabolism of lipids in the body. This puts hemp seed oil right in the forefront of known oils. It contains a wealth of valuable components. In its composition it has 25 times more omega-3 oil and 40 percent less saturated fat than olive oil.

One tablespoon contains:

Linolenic Acid (omega-6)	56.77%
Alpha Linolenic Acid (omega-3)	18.33%
Oleic Acid (omega-9)	10.32%
Palmitic Acid	5.79%
Gamma Linolenic Acid (omega-6)	3.98%
Stearic Acid	2.28%
Steridonic Acid (omega-3)	1.18%

Hemp seed oil has a chemical composition very similar to the natural oil created by the human skin. Creams, lotions and other cosmetics containing this oil are very well accepted by the skin, and it is especially good for conditions like acne, seborrhoea and enlarged pores. Problems like eczema and psoriasis are substantially mitigated.

Hemp seed oil is a treasure trove of vitamin K, which is essential for the synthesis of proteins and enzymes. This vitamin is known for its anti-hemorrhagic properties and is responsible for healthy blood-clotting.

This oil has a very effective anti-allergic effect. It also has the ability to assist in skin regeneration, stimulating it and improving its appearance, making it a great anti-aging agent.

The hemp plants themselves have an extremely beneficial effect on the soil. Depending on the type of soil, their strong roots bind or loosen the soil beneficially. The roots remaining after felling contain many nutrients that nourish the soil and improve soil fertility, making it ideal for crop rotation programmes.

Hemp also has a valuable property through which it draws heavy metals and toxic substances from the soil. This makes it ideal for cleaning contaminated sites. It also absorbs a lot of carbon dioxide during growth thereby improving the air quality. All of these properties make industrial hemp one of the most environmentally friendly and useful plants in the world.

Scientific studies have shown that the extracted hemp seed oil contains no psychoactive substances or residual substances that are potentially harmful to human skin. Pure hemp seed oil can be applied directly to the skin without any adverse effects.

Cold pressed hemp seed oil has excellent nutritional properties. It is also anti-allergic, regenerative, anti-aging as well as emollient. Chlorophyll, which causes the slightly green tint of the oil, works as a soothing anti-inflammatory agent.

It doesn't take a genius to figure out that Mother Nature provides the perfect food and medicine for our bodies. No human concoction can match a product like hemp. You can and will live longer and healthier and enjoy much improved energy levels if you use products derived from this plant. When I discovered and started using the seeds and the oil, available from health shops, I could hardly believe the powerful effects of this amazing plant. Since then I have become obsessed with this plant. I am convinced that even my memory has improved since I have been using it.

This book is about health and if you want to be slim and healthy you need to give your body the right nutrients so that you can stop being hungry between meals. Our brains need omega-3 and omega-6 in the correct balance to function properly and make good decisions. Consuming hemp seeds and hemp seed oil can greatly help you in this regard.

Unfortunately most people only know about this plant because it is labelled as a drug-producing plant; everyone has heard of cannabis and marijuana. By abusing this wonderfully powerful plant you can cause your body to experience a so-called 'high' from the THC contained in the plant. However, this is a matter of choice: you will not get high from using hemp products if you don't want to. You can use this plant for its amazing medicinal and nutritional value with a clear conscience.

It is clear to see what happens to animals when their diet is lacking the right balance of nutrients.

I would like to see more crop rotation being practised in agriculture, especially with plants like hemp, to improve the quality of our soil and our food, which for me is very important.

Before you can lose weight, you need to concentrate on eating foods that will provide your body with the right amount of nutrients. By doing so, you will automatically experience less cravings for junk food. You won't need to cram large volumes of food into your stomach to feel satisfied. You will lose weight naturally and efficiently. The entire process will not be an ordeal. Losing excessive weight can be a pleasant, natural experience. Remember, just as it takes time to gain weight, so too it takes time to lose weight.

If you like, you can go on a hemp fast for one day, consuming the seeds and the oil and nothing else. This will give your body an amazing energy boost, cleanse your digestive system and shrink your stomach.

We all know products like alcohol and cigarettes are bad for you. But that does not mean that the plants used to make them are bad. We don't ban tobacco plants because they are bad, so why should we do so with hemp? Mother Nature does not create products that are harmful – it is we humans who abuse the power of nature.

Why did nature create such a wonderful plant that is so easy to grow if we cannot use it? It has so many useful applications. Hemp fibre is better than cotton, it is easier to grow and needs no pesticides, yet we continue to use cotton. Maybe it's time to re-evaluate the advantages of this amazing plant. It is cheap, simple to grow and offers much value.

Plants can't speak for themselves, but I can. That's why I feature this plant so prominently in my book. Do people marginalise this plant because it is so much better than its competitors?

I strongly recommend the nutritional and medicinal properties of hemp. Visit your local health store and try out the seeds and the oil. You will be pleasantly surprised!

Another one of my favourite natural products, derived from the flax plant, is ***linseed oil***.

The history of flax cultivation also dates back thousands of years. The first documented reports of the healing properties of flax date back to about 650 BC. Later on Hippocrates advocated the use of flax for inflammation of the mucous membranes as well as for various abdominal ailments.

The late Mahatma Gandhi remarked: "Wherever flax seed is regularly consumed, people enjoy better health".

Cold pressed linseed oil has a distinctive smell, a yellow colour and a slightly nutty taste. The omega-3 in linseed oil is fundamental to the functioning of our bodies, acting among others as the building blocks for brain tissue, hormones and every cell in the body.

The proper balance of omega-3 and omega-6 oil intake protects against premature birth. A deficiency of these fatty acids cause changes in the cell membranes of the brain and retina.

Breast milk is a very rich source of these acids, which are necessary for the proper development of the brain and nervous system of a developing child. Of course, the level of these acids depends on the foods consumed by a mother. Deficiency of these nutrients is said to result in skin lesions, reduced resistance to infections and inferior physical development.

Linseed oil is good for the health of children and youths and aids the proper development of neurons.

It prevents and helps in the treatment of hyperactivity (ADHD) and promotes hormonal balance, reducing acne.

It is good for adult women too. Linseed oil is beneficial for regulating the menstrual cycle and helps to alleviate the symptoms associated with menstruation. It also alleviates the symptoms of menopause and promotes uterine activity.

Men also need linseed oil. It can treat infertility and reduce the risk of prostate diseases.

This product is excellent in promoting mental health. It supports the treatment of depression and the production of beneficial hormones like serotonin and dopamine in the right quantities.

Linseed oil also converts nutrients for energy for people dedicated to sport. It promotes muscle growth and fat reduction. It is also involved in the transport of oxygen in the blood, ultimately benefiting cell regeneration.

Alpha-linolenic acid (ALA) is the primary source of DHA as a very important component of the brain. Low levels of DHA are associated with mood changes, memory loss, problems with vision and the occurrence of neurological disorders.

Linseed oil helps to restore hormonal balance by changing the proportions of fatty acids in the body. Because of its therapeutic properties, linseed oil is sometimes used in therapeutic massage of the skin, feeding it and giving it flexibility.

In addition, linseed oil contains vitamin E, called the vitamin of youth; it protects the skin from premature aging. It also prevents the formation of blackheads.

Only cold linseed oil should be consumed. Do not heat it. Store it in a cold, dark place, preferably in the fridge. Heating and exposure to light and air reduces its efficacy.

It is best served as an addition to salads, vegetables, soups, or used on bread instead of butter.

It is important to use linseed oil as quickly as possible – within a month. Check the expiry date. Nutritionists emphasize that 'broken' linseed oil is a known carcinogen.

A final word on flax seeds. When I was a child my mother used to boil flax seeds in water for a few minutes (one tablespoon in half a litre = 2 cups of water), stirring all the time up to 10 minutes, until it became a gel. This gel is a wonderful food for when you have an upset stomach. There is no better medicine for diarrhoea or nausea. You can use it for small children and elderly people, or you can simply just eat it to make your stomach stronger. This is just one of many potent natural remedies that modern society has forgotten about.

Now I would like to introduce you to another one of my favourite natural products, namely *coconut oil.*

As I write this, coconut products are rapidly becoming very popular. Of course, coconut is very tasty and as an added bonus it contains vitamins B2, B6, C and E, as well as folic acid, potassium, calcium, magnesium, phosphorous, iron, sodium and zinc.

Scientific analysis has shown that the juice inside a coconut is in many ways almost identical to the composition of human blood plasma. During World War II it was successfully used a fluid transfusion when blood ran out. Coconut water readily mixes with blood and is rapidly absorbed by the human body. In some under-developed countries it is used intravenously in the form of drips to supplement electrolyte deficiency.

It must, however, be used directly from the fruit to maintain its sterility.

Coconut juice is one of the richest sources of electrolytes. It contains more of them than most sports drinks used by athletes. It also contains more potassium than bananas. It is recommended for diarrhoea, vomiting and stomach problems.

Coconut oil is sold in two forms. The regular, refined form is readily available, but the cold pressed version is quite rare. The cold pressed oil retains the typical, natural coconut smell and taste and is a very valuable and sought-after product. The refined version is almost odourless.

Coconut oil has a variety of uses: it can be used in the kitchen as well as for medicinal purposes.

Due to its solid form it is suitable as an oil spread and can also be used to replace butter in baking. It is ideal for frying at high temperatures, it does not smoke, it does not become rancid, and thanks to its unique characteristics it flavours food with its universally loved taste and aroma.

This oil contains practically no fatty acids that can oxidise, which makes it very stable during cooking at high temperatures, making it much healthier to use than many of the more common oils. Not many people know that oils such as soybean, sunflower or groundnut oil should not be heated to high temperatures.

I once heard the story of a lady who would always cut off a small portion of a leg of lamb before putting it into a large pot to roast it. When her husband asked her why she did this, she said it was because her mother always did it. The husband was curious though and got his wife to phone her mother to ask her why she cut a portion off the leg of lamb before pot-roasting it. Strangely enough, the lady's mother said she didn't know either – her own mother always used to do it too. Fortunately the grandmother was still alive, so they phoned her up to find out why she always cut off a portion of the lamb before roasting it. "Well that's easy to answer" the grandmother replied, "In those days I always cut off a piece of the lamb because it didn't fit into my pot!"

Perhaps we can all learn a lesson from this simple story.
Coconut oil is also the first fat that does not contribute to the manufacture of body fat; on the contrary, it stimulates metabolism and actually promotes weight loss.

Lauric acid is found in nature in large amounts only in coconut and in breast milk. Coconut oil helps strengthen immunity, demonstrating strong anti-bacterial, anti-fungal and anti-viral properties. Lauric acid in particular is well suited to fight infections, rashes and eczema, as well as contributing to the treatment of minor cuts and micro-traumas in the skin. It also reduces itching and the pain of insect bites.

Coconut oil contains natural antioxidants that fight free radicals, slowing the aging process of the skin, making it become firmer and more elastic.

This oil has also become very popular in cosmetics. The oil moisturises the skin of the whole body. It is the only oil that protects the hair from losing protein. Due to it specific composition coconut oil is able to penetrate into the hair and moisten it thoroughly, making hair soft, shiny and strong.

For decades this foodstuff was condemned as it was thought the content of saturated fatty acids caused the development of diseases like obesity, heart attacks and atherosclerosis. However, Pacific Islanders who eat coconuts in large quantities daily are proof of the inaccuracy of this theory. They are generally slim and enjoy glowing health.

Fortunately, Western consumers are now discovering the multiple benefits and positive qualities of coconut products for themselves.

Kefir is a fermented milk product that originated centuries ago in the Caucasus Mountains, and is now enjoyed by many different cultures worldwide, particularly in Europe and Asia. It can be made from the milk of any ruminant animal, such as cows, goats, or sheep. It is slightly sour and carbonated due to the fermentation activity of the symbiotic colony of bacteria and yeast that make up the "grains" used to culture the milk (not actual grains, but a grain-like matrix of proteins, lipids, and sugars that feed the microbes). **The various types of beneficial**

bacteria contained in kefir make it one of the most potent probiotic foods available.

Besides containing highly beneficial bacteria and yeasts, kefir is a rich source of many different vitamins, minerals and essential amino acids that promote healing and repair, as well as general health maintenance. Kefir contains high levels of thiamin, B12, calcium and vitamin K2. It is a good source of biotin, a B vitamin that helps the body to assimilate other B vitamins. The complete proteins in kefir are already partially digested, and are therefore more easily utilized by the body. Like many other dairy products, kefir is a great source of minerals like calcium and magnesium, as well as phosphorus, which helps the body utilize carbohydrates, fats and proteins for cell growth, maintenance and energy.

Also known as Tibetan mushroom, kefir is a potent probiotic, consisting of both bacterial and yeast species of beneficial flora, and helps protect against gastrointestinal diseases. It has also been demonstrated to improve lactose digestion in adults with lactose intolerance. In addition to providing the gut with healthy symbiotic micro-flora, many studies have also demonstrated the anti-fungal and antibacterial properties of kefir. Certain bacteria strains from the kefir culture have been shown to help in treating colitis by regulating the inflammatory response of the intestinal cells.

As the kefir deconstructs the milk it is placed in, it consumes the sugar in the milk and turns it into lactic acid. As a result it removes just about all the lactose, making it suitable for people who are lactose intolerant.

You can order kefir grains (also called Tibetan mushroom) on the internet along with simple instructions on how to make your own at home. In my experience I found it to be a great help in losing weight and boosting energy. As my kefir grains have developed and multiplied, I have passed them on to many of my friends and they all rave about the wonderful properties of this 'super food'. Many people claim that it has cured them of all sorts of diseases and it definitely helps to curb hunger pangs.

Kefir is unrivalled for attaining and maintaining healthy functioning of your digestive tract and helps you to manage your stomach volume. I strongly recommend it.

In conclusion, here is something that everyone should try – *oil pulling*.

In recent times people have rediscovered a technique that is described in Ayurvedic literature. I practise oil pulling myself and have found it to be extremely beneficial to my health.

Oil pulling heals headaches, bronchitis, asthma, toothache, thrombosis, eczema, ulcers and diseases of the stomach, intestines, heart, blood, kidney, liver, lungs and women's diseases. It heals diseases of nerves, chronic sleeplessness, paralysis and encephalitis. It prevents the growth of malignant tumours and also speeds up the healing process of cuts.

You have doubtless seen little children sucking on their thumbs. This reflex is provided by nature as part of the child's self-preservation instinct. Its task is to produce large amounts of saliva, which has an anti-bacterial effect. This is probably where folk medicine got the idea for a therapy which uses a similar mechanism – holding vegetable oil in the mouth for up to 30 minutes produces a proven therapeutic effect.

The amount of blood circulating our mouth area in 30 minutes equals around four litres. Because vegetable oil has good absorbing qualities, this method uses these qualities to absorb toxic substances from our bodies.

How to do oil pulling?

First thing in the morning, on an empty stomach, before drinking any liquids (including water), pour exactly one tablespoon of sunflower, sesame or coconut oil into your mouth. My own preference is coconut oil.

Swish the oil around in your mouth without swallowing it. Move it around in your mouth and through your teeth, as if it were mouthwash. You'll find that the oil becomes watery as your saliva mixes with it. Keep swishing. If your jaw muscles get sore while swishing, you are putting too much effort into it. Relax your jaw muscles and use your tongue to help move the liquid around in your mouth.

When you do this correctly you will soon feel very comfortable. There is no right way or wrong way to swish and pull oil. Don't focus on doing it right. Do it with a very natural movement: gently, not vigorously, in a relaxed way for about 20 minutes. I always take a shower while doing this and time just flies!

It might be a bit unpleasant at first when you're not used to it, but soon after it won't be bothersome at all and will be as simple as brushing your teeth.

When the oil becomes saturated with the toxins it has pulled out, it may become whitish and have a thinner milky consistency, depending on the type of oil used. Each time you oil pull, it can take a different amount of time to reach that state, so 20 minutes is a general rule of thumb, but you can experiment with this.

As the end of the oil pulling session approaches, spit the oil out into the toilet then rinse the mouth with warm salt water. Salt water rinsing isn't absolutely necessary, but it is helpful as an anti-microbial wash to soothe any inflammation and it is proven to be effective in rinsing out any toxins which may be left in your mouth.

Eventually you will start to feel the difference: you will feel refreshed, energetic and calm. Acute diseases are cured quickly – within two to three weeks. Chronic conditions may take several months to a year and you should be aware that the therapy might trigger certain mild symptoms (e.g. the feeling of weakness) during the first week. This phenomenon is associated with the weakening of the disease's focal points. It is normal and we need to go through the experience.

Properly implemented therapy will bring noticeable signs such as more energy on awakening, better appetite, and the feeling of freshness. Based on the state of your health you can make your own decision about the duration of the therapy. This will not only prevent diseases mentioned above, but will also remove toxic heavy metals that can be found even in a healthy body. Regular oil pulling also reduces snoring.

You can do the oil pulling every morning or several times a week. I do it daily. One immediate benefit of this method is that everyone gets whiter teeth – I could see a difference after only one week. After a week my skin also looked fresh and glowed like never before!

Healthy people and children can use this method too. Oil pulling not only cures but also prevents diseases. This method is really simple, painless and absolutely harmless and I think it is well worth a try.

Lemon water and pH balance

Many health experts now believe that our pH balance is extremely important to sustain good health. Studies show that most people are too acidic; ideally our pH should be slightly alkaline. Apart from our stomachs, which naturally are acidic to aid in the digestion of food, our bodies – tissue, muscle, organs, cells, bones and blood – are more susceptible to inflammation and harmful pathogens in an acidic environment.

So how does the body become acidic? Through unbalanced diets too rich in acid-producing or inflammatory foods, repressed emotions, negative subconscious thought patterns and overall wear and tear in human body functions.

One of the best ways to rectify your pH balance over time is by drinking a glass of warm water with the juice of half a lemon every morning. This may sound strange to you, as we all know that lemon, being a citrus fruit, is acidic. However, once the lemon has been fully metabolised inside your body and the minerals are dissociated in your bloodstream, its effect is alkalising and therefore raises the pH of the body (pH above 7 is alkaline).

Of course, lemon juice is also a rich source of nutrients like calcium, potassium, vitamin C and pectin fibre. It also has various medicinal values and antibacterial properties and contains traces of iron and vitamin A.

Lemon undoubtedly helps maintain your immune system and thus protects you from most types of infections. It also plays the role of a blood purifier.

Lemon juice flushes out unwanted materials and toxins from the body. Its atomic composition is similar to saliva and the hydrochloric acid of digestive juices. It encourages the liver to produce bile which is an acid that is required for digestion. The digestive qualities of lemon juice help to relieve symptoms of indigestion, such as heartburn, belching and bloating. The American Cancer Society actually recommends offering warm lemon water to cancer sufferers to help stimulate bowel movements.

Boosts Your Immune System. Lemons are high in vitamin C, which is great for fighting colds. They're high in potassium, which stimulates brain and nerve function. Potassium also helps control blood pressure. Ascorbic acid (vitamin C) found in lemons demonstrates anti-inflammatory effects, and is used as complementary support for asthma and other respiratory symptoms plus it enhances iron absorption in the body; iron plays an important role in immune function. Lemons also contain saponins, which show antimicrobial properties that may help keep cold and flu at bay. Lemons also reduce the amount of phlegm produced by the body.

Balances pH Levels. Lemons are one of the most alkalizing foods for the body. The juice contains both citric and ascorbic acid, weak acids easily metabolized in the body allowing the mineral content of lemons to help alkalize the blood. Disease states only occur when the body pH is acidic. Drinking lemon water regularly can help to remove overall acidity in the body, including uric acid in the joints.

Clears Skin. The vitamin C component as well as other antioxidants helps decrease wrinkles and blemishes and it helps to combat free radical damage. Vitamin C is vital for healthy glowing skin while its alkaline nature kills some types of bacteria known to cause acne.

It can actually be applied directly to scars or age spots to help reduce their appearance. Since lemon water purges toxins from your blood, it would also be helping to keep your skin clear of blemishes from the inside out. The vitamin C contained in the lemon rejuvenates the skin from within your body.

Energizes You and Enhances Your Mood. The energy you receive from food comes from the atoms and molecules in your food. A reaction occurs when the positively charged ions from food enter the digestive tract and interact with the negatively charged enzymes. Lemon is one of the few foods that contain more negatively charged ions, providing your body with more energy when it enters the digestive tract.

Promotes Healing. Ascorbic acid (vitamin C), found in abundance in lemons, promotes wound healing, and is an essential nutrient in the maintenance of healthy bones, connective tissue, and cartilage. As noted previously, vitamin C also displays anti-inflammatory properties. Combined, vitamin C is an essential nutrient in the maintenance of good health and recovery from stress and injury.

Aids in Weight Loss. Lemons are high in pectin fiber, which helps fight hunger cravings. Studies have shown people who maintain a more alkaline diet, do in fact lose weight faster. I personally find myself making better choices throughout the day, if I start my day off right, by making a health conscious choice to drink warm lemon water first thing every morning.

So, do you really want to be slim and healthy? Would you like to have more energy and a brighter outlook on life? Then please focus on natural foods and natural products that have proved their worth to humans over thousands of years.

I sincerely hope you enjoy the process of losing weight and discovering a new zest for life. Don't rush the process. Take your time. If you combine good eating habits with some healthy exercise you will see faster, more dramatic results. I wish you all the best on this exciting journey you are about to take and remember, nobody but you can control your future. Enjoy it!

To summarise:

- Hemp, linseed and coconut oil are powerful agents for good health.
- Give yourself a daily dose of one or two tablespoons of these oils – you can pour it on salad or even on bread.
- Oil pulling is an excellent way to detoxify your body and is really good for healthy joints.
- Hemp and flax seeds are also very beneficial for animals.
- Lemon water is very good to adjust the pH balance in your body.

These natural oils, or super fuels as I like to call them, are easy to use and produce astonishing results for good health.

Chapter 5

Where do I start?

For most people it is really difficult to lose weight and very easy to gain weight. I truly sympathise with the poor souls who have struggled with this issue for so many years. How fortunate I was, as a young girl, to discover the article about the scientist who experimented on feeding rats. I believe that lead me to the secret of solving this vexing problem.

Maybe this book will allow you to turn the corner once and for all. Your body needs real food to function properly. By real food I mean real nutrients, not just tasty bulk that will fill your stomach but fail to feed your body.

Keep in mind that we are all different. Just as we are different in appearance, we are different on the inside. So for me to tell you to do exactly what I do might not work so well for you. That's the reason why some diets work for some people but fail for others. You need to grasp the essence and the importance of eating the right food and then you can start experimenting with what works best for your own body.

Please don't accept the 'fact' that you are fat and there is nothing you can do about it.

Forty years ago when I was 'hopelessly' fat, eating too much processed food and too little fresh, live food, I somehow knew that I was doing something wrong on a very basic level. When I read about how well the rats fared on fresh food in that scientific experiment, the lights went on for me.

I started to experiment with different foods and I soon realised that processed food and over-cooked food did my body no good whatsoever. It had nothing to do with hormones or genes or a big bone structure. It had everything to do with what I put into my mouth every day.

Once you understand the basic premise of good nutrition, your first priority is to start controlling the volume of your stomach. By eating the right foods, you will be satisfied sooner and for much longer and your overall health will benefit as well.

Start with fresh food. Mother Nature produces exactly what your body needs, and she has a huge variety to choose from. It is your privilege and your pleasure to try out these different offerings and to see which ones work best for you. Soon you will find that there is a large portion of the supermarket, that does not sell fresh food, that you simply ignore – like I do all the time. You will be shopping in that part of the store that sells fresh, live food; food that truly nourishes your body.

I recently observed two girls in their twenties in my local supermarket, both were overweight and clearly had too much abdominal fat (this is quite common nowadays). They were buying food for lunch (I couldn't help overhearing them): fried chicken, potato crisps, pies and chocolate. From their conversation I could hear that the girls both honestly believed that these were healthy foods. I was astonished by their ignorance.

At the time of writing this book more and more scientific studies are emerging that prove processed food and especially sugar cause diabetes (usually type 2 diabetes). In many cases the diabetes goes undetected, but it triggers a whole variety of destructive ailments including high blood pressure and heart disease. Invariably it goes hand in hand with obesity.

Avoid food with preservatives. Our bodies don't have the enzymes to cope with preservatives. Sometimes even semi-prepared fruit and vegetables (peeled and sliced), that have been attractively packaged, have been treated with preservatives. It's best to buy raw and cut and slice at home.

In the 1990s the word went out that plastic cutting boards in the kitchen were much safer than wooden boards. Well, this theory has now been proven incorrect. Microbiologists now agree that wooden cutting boards harbour far less bacteria than plastic or even glass or marble boards. The best and safest wooden cutting boards, apparently, are made from oak, beech or bamboo. The best way to clean these boards are with salt or baking soda, which are more natural than detergents.

When I started my fresh food diet 40 years ago, I didn't go to the gym because it was not a popular thing to do in those days. Also, I had not yet discovered the many benefits of exercise. However, I did walk a lot and that certainly helped, but a regular exercise routine will definitely shape and rejuvenate your body in a very short time.

All these years I have been observing people eat bad food and getting stuck in a sedentary lifestyle. Most of them have weight problems and suffering from disorders like diabetes and high blood pressure. These problems are rapidly on the increase today. As a result, many people are on chronic medication for the rest of their lives. Lately I have also seen an increase in obesity in children and young adults. Who makes them fat? Their bodies were not designed to be obese. To add to these woes, these people are chronically sick and in many cases they are desperately unhappy and even depressed. The root cause is eating the wrong food.

If you look at nature you'll see no obese wild animals. That's because they eat and exercise in accordance with the way they were designed.

Forget about counting calories. It's a really stupid weight loss technique. Eat fresh, live food and do some exercise every day and you can eat as much as you like until you are satisfied – within reason of course (remember the 1.5 litre ice cream container). That's the way your body was made. That's the real you!

If you are overweight, your stomach has probably expanded. When I was a fat 16 year-old I could eat two litres of ice cream and I didn't even feel full. My stomach was enlarged. Fortunately our stomachs have the capacity to shrink to the correct size if we eat properly. How many people regularly eat too much of the wrong food, especially deep-fried and over-processed food from restaurants and fast food establishments?

I have seen farmers work at expanding the stomach of animals so they can grow quickly and be sold sooner. In France they used to force feed geese to get them fat quickly so their livers would eventually also be enlarged. The poor birds were so fat they could hardly walk properly. The same has been done to pigs. These animals would get sick very easily and they would have to be given antibiotics quite frequently.

Another way to take good care of your stomach is to regularly take natural probiotics in the form of yogurt or kefir. These foods promote a healthy digestive system and boost your immune system. They also undo the damage done by antibiotics, which kill the good bacteria in your stomach. Both yoghurt and kefir can be made at home, and I encourage you to do so.

Apart from being bad for your digestive system, alcohol has a long list of detrimental effects on your body. Some people take alcohol socially and some take it to reduce stress. Of course, it actually causes a lot of stress in the long run. The relaxed feeling you get from a drink is very temporary. Invariably you pay a heavy price for it. You experience the same food poisoning symptoms that you would get from eating not-so-fresh chicken or fish. Have you seen how nauseous people can get when they've been on a drinking binge?

I suppose I don't need to give you a lecture on the evils of alcohol – they are well known. Suffice to say that alcohol, and especially distilled alcohol, is not good for you at all.

Very few people have the self discipline to drink only one glass of wine a day, so I'm not even going to get into the supposed benefits of a little red wine. Yes, I know the resveratrol in red wine has certain benefits, but you can buy resveratrol supplements from your health store if you really want it. Alcohol is addictive and undoubtedly fattening as well, so that's a good enough reason to cut down and even abstain from taking it. Make the right choice!

As a young adult I used to consume alcohol, but I soon realised that it has no benefits whatsoever. I'm not against people enjoying their lives and getting jolly once in a while; I'm just pointing out that alcohol works against all the good intentions you have for your own personal health and wellbeing. It has the potential to literally poison and damage your body, to make you appear stupid, to make you fat, as well as to cause chronic depression and a host of other mental, physical and social disorders. Exercise will give you a better, longer-lasting good mood. Instead of going to the pub after work, go to the gym!

As you embark on this journey of changing your lifestyle by making a few simple choices, you will soon start seeing amazing results. These results will motivate you to keep going. You will feel better and better as every day goes by and then you'll be even more motivated. The secret lies in getting started.

Your body and your health is in your own hands. Take a photo of yourself right now and as you take charge of your life by taking the advice in this book you can take photos of yourself as you progress. This will also help to keep you motivated. To be slim and healthy has always been my goal.

If you give a potted plant the right ingredients of sun, water and good soil it flourishes. However, if you take that plant and place it in a dark room, it would still continue to develop and grow very slowly. After a while, though, it will start to deteriorate. Then if you put it back in its preferred environment it will start to grow vigorously again. People respond in the same way. If humans eat, sleep and exercise well, they will flourish. Some people are often ill because they deviate from these requirements. But if they change this unhealthy pattern, like the plant they will start to flourish again. Are you like a wilting plant?

The improvement in your general health, losing weight naturally, increased energy levels and reduced stress levels should be more than enough to make you happy, right? Why would you ever want to go back to your old lifestyle? When you experience real good health, you won't turn back; in fact, you will go out of your way to convince your family and friends of these benefits.

Strangely enough, people always want the recipe of a tasty dish, but they hardly ever ask for the 'recipe' of lasting good health.

Being a fat young girl was the worst time in my life. Because I struggled with this issue and have subsequently found the simple, natural and obvious secret to becoming and staying slim and healthy, I would dearly like you to enjoy this wonderful freedom and happiness too. You will also find that people call you lucky.

Maybe you need to develop a new routine in your life. Forming new habits takes only a few days of persistence; and it starts by making a good quality decision. Once you have a set routine, the results will keep you motivated going forward. Once you have a set routine, you can keep it for the rest of your life.

Your body is an incredible machine. Nothing man has ever made can match it. By simply treating your body wisely you can restore your health. Remember the wilting plant? Like most things in life (e.g. your car, your house etc.) your body needs to be diligently maintained to keep it in good condition. Your body needs the right treatment. Your body can even cope with years of abuse, but after a while it will let you know that it can only take so much. We were made to eat fresh, natural food. It's as simple as that. Maybe it is because it is so simple that people have overlooked it.

As people get older they actually expect that they will start to develop diseases and disorders. This will certainly come to pass if they have been practising the wrong lifestyle all their lives. There is more than enough proof, however, that you can have a slim, fit and healthy body even in your old age – sometimes even better than young people who abuse their bodies.

It's not a question of luck or good genes. How you treat your body has a telling effect on how your body will treat you. Food is not your enemy; the *wrong food* is your enemy. Your body needs fresh, live food all the time. It's okay to love food; I certainly do! Just stick to my recipe of eating good, natural food – preferably organic – and don't over-extend your stomach.

Talking of organic, it's time we supported the farmers who produce nutrient-rich, pesticide-free organic food.

Eat good food and your body will produce enough energy to exercise. By exercising you will increase your oxygen intake, tone your muscles and reduce your stress. With less stress and a healthy, better-looking body you'll be so much happier. Can I put it any simpler?

How would I go about starting a new lifestyle?

As I've said before, everyone is different. Also, everyone has differing circumstances so I can and will not be prescriptive as to how you should start out with a new eating plan. Having read the book this far, I am sure you will already have a good idea of how you want to start out.

However, many people ask me for more specific information. To satisfy these people I'm going to give you a few pointers, but I stress once again: use the ones that you are comfortable with. As long as you stick to the basic guidelines of eating good, natural, live food and doing some beneficial exercise at least five times a week, you are already on the right track.

This is my suggested starting regime designed to shrink your stomach, boost your energy and get you losing weight immediately:

- After waking, I suggest 10 – 20 minutes of oil-pulling (I prefer coconut oil). Do this for a few weeks.
- Make yourself a glass of warm water with freshly squeezed lemon. Do this for a few weeks. I suggest you alternate this with oil-pulling.
- Drink freshly squeezed juice (I suggest carrots and apples along with any of your favourites) interchangeably with a little water throughout the day. Prepare the juice beforehand. You need at least two litres of fluid a day. So, for example, a litre of juice and a litre of water.
- Go to the gym, preferably on an empty stomach (before or after work).
- After exercise eat mainly live, organic food like meat, lightly grilled steak, steak tartare, fish, turkey, boiled eggs, fruit and almonds, as much as you want (without stretching your stomach).

- During the day you can snack on almonds or seeds, preferably hemp (shelled or unshelled) or you can add them to yogurt or salad.
- Take two tablespoons of oil (hemp, coconut or flax; straight-up or poured on bread or salad). Buy small containers and finish the oil soon; the fresher, the better. Check the expiry date.
- Take approximately 200 ml of kefir or real yoghurt before going to bed.
- If you have to drink tea or coffee during the day, avoid sugar or sweeteners.
- Food prepared at home can be lightly grilled, steamed or boiled (but not fried!) – you don't need to cook so much – keep it simple.
- Everything in nature, from a flower to a snowflake, is unique. No two are exactly the same. So too with humans; even identical twins are unique individuals. You are a unique individual, so find out what works best for you!

This entire regime is for optimal results, so I don't expect you to necessarily follow it all religiously from day one.

Remember, you are about to make an important, life-enhancing lifestyle change. That means you are going to form new habits. By doing so, old habits will fall away naturally. It's a bit like learning to drive a car: the first few efforts may cause a little tension and stuttering, but you'll soon get the hang of it. The more you do it, the better you become at doing it.

Habit forming is connected to yourself image and yourself belief. Convince yourself that you are doing something that will dramatically change your life for the better. Visualise yourself as slim and healthy with a lot of energy all the time. Everything starts with a thought. If you can win the battle between your ears, you are half way to victory.

I realise that much of the information in this book is not new to you. It may even sound a little old-fashioned, but I can assure you it really works. Be patient. Set yourself small goals and just keep at it. A slow and steady approach is always sensible. Don't despair if you are not losing kilograms or centimetres from the outset. Sometimes your body just needs time to adjust to a new routine. Soon your new routine will become your new 'normal'. Don't give up – this is the one battle that is really worth fighting.

Can you do it? Of course you can! The only question is: do you really want to? If the desire is strong enough you cannot fail. By taking the first step, then the next one, and the next one, you are on your way. Nothing can stop you now!

I wish you all the very best as you embark on this most exciting journey. Like I did, you can change your life forever; one step at a time and one day at a time. Before you know it, people will hardly recognise you because you look so fabulously slim and attractive. You will just laugh when people talk about this diet and that diet. Who needs a diet if you know the secret to a truly natural, healthy lifestyle?

* * *

Like energy, nutrition is a vital feature of all living organisms and constitutes one of the most important laws of nature. This law states that whatever we consume should be filled with natural energy. Man-made medications are devoid of such power and contain hardly any substances beneficial to human beings. Living creatures can be helped only by living nature. The healing power of an organism can only be aided by the healing power of life that comes from nature. We eat to live. Living is acquiring energy. In order to live humans need to acquire energy from the four basic elements that sustain the existence of all organisms on Earth.

These are the elements which the ancient philosophers regarded as the source of everything in the universe, namely earth, water, fire and air. In order to live, our bodies need only those products which contain these elements. Those products which don't have them are empty and even harmful. Where is the energy source of fire? In the sun. All produce grown in sunshine is filled with the energy of fire, including grains, fruits, vegetables, nuts, seeds, green leaves and bulb and root plants. When a green leaf absorbs sunlight it assimilates the energy of the sun and, of course, the energy of life. The energy of the sun is best preserved in those products that haven't undergone heat treatment. In the same way, all plants that grow in the open air are filled with the energy of the air.

Water is an inseparable part of any living organism. Similarly, it is impossible to obtain real life energy without consuming energy from the Earth. The Earth is the source of important and beneficial minerals and micro-elements in the precise form and composition needed in the human body. So only what grows out of the Earth is beneficial to human beings.

Please remember this: natural principles promote life!

God bless you!

www.ingramcontent.com/pod-product-compliance
Lightning Source LLC
Chambersburg PA
CBHW070800010626
R18376100001B/R183761PG45790CBX00020B/7